MW00723680

The Older I Get, the Less I Care

Teresa Roberts Logan

**Andrews McMeel
Publishing, LLC**

Kansas City

The Older I Get, the Less I Care

08 09 10 11 12 TWP 10 9 8 7 6 5 4 3 2 1

ISBN-13: 978-0-7407-7114-9

ISBN-10: 0-7407-7114-0

Library of Congress Control Number: 2007933993

www.andrewsmcmeel.com

ATTENTION: SCHOOLS AND BUSINESSES
Andrews McMeel books are available at quantity discounts with bulk purchase for educational, business, or sales promotional use. For information, please write to: Special Sales Department, Andrews McMeel Publishing, LLC, 4520 Main Street, Kansas City, Missouri 64111.

This book is dedicated to women everywhere,
because we all need laughter
and encouragement.

It is especially dedicated to my mom, "Betty
Jean the Beauty Queen," who, along with my
dad, taught me to laugh in the first place.

Special thanks to Patricia Rice, and to my
awesome husband, Gary, and my wonderful
son, Andrew; thanks for always believing in
me and for laughing at my "stuff."

The Older I Get, the Less I Care

. . . about objects in the mirror being
LARGER than they appear.

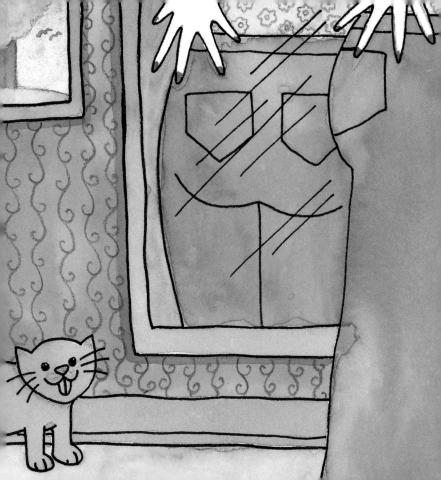

. . . about who got plastic surgery . . .
and who's for real!

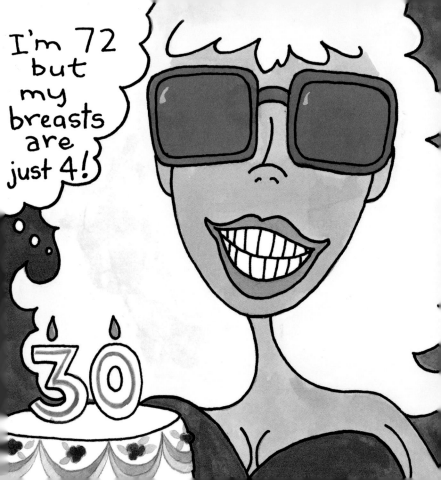

. . . about the sociological implications
of my shoe fetish.

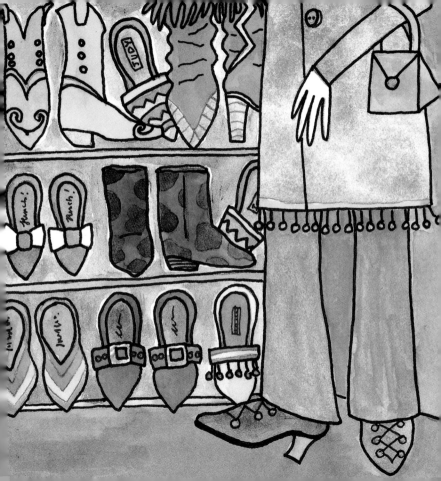

. . . about stifling my big, LOUD laugh!

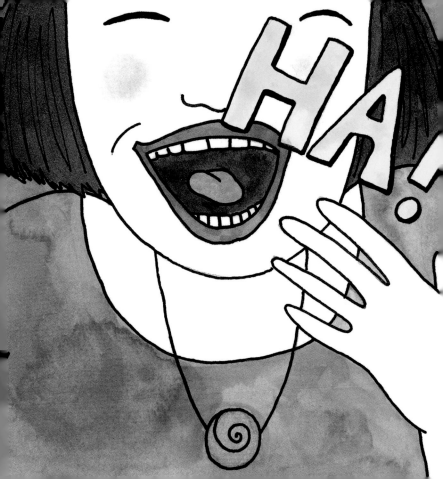

. . . about my fear of clowns.

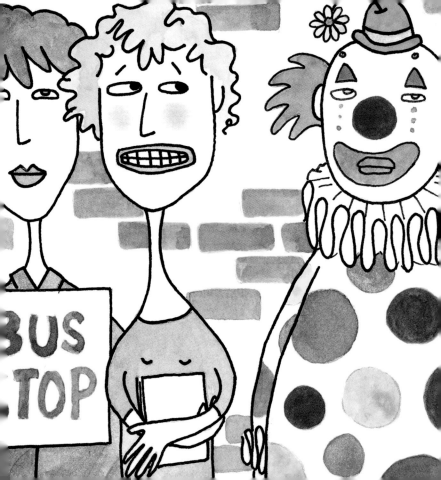

. . . about liking my pets too much.

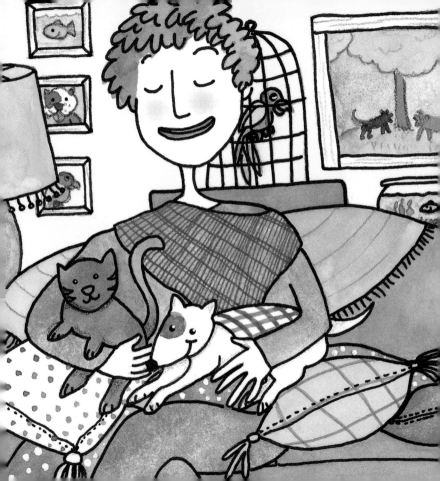

. . . about the difference
ONE dessert makes!

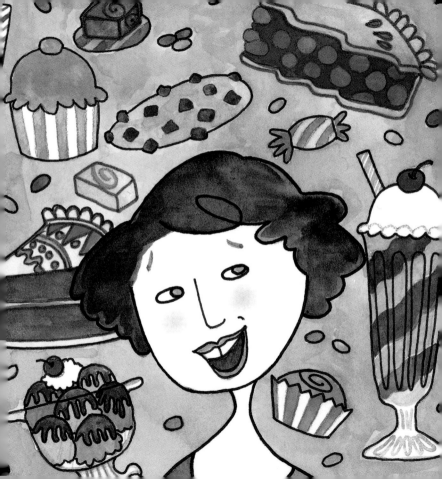

. . . about whether my clothes
are too loud!

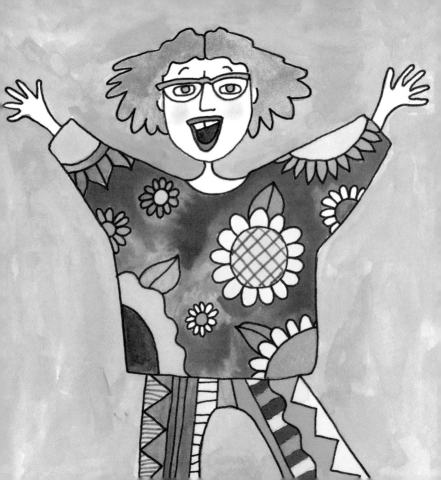

. . . about sounding hip!

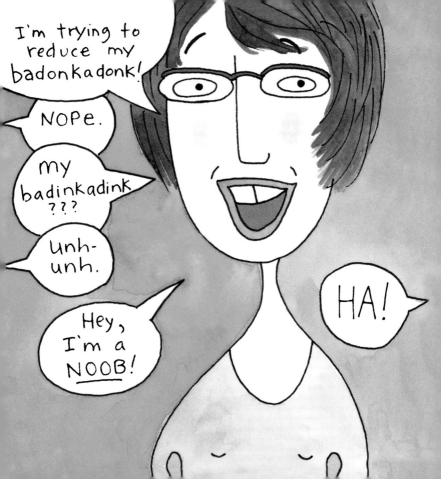

. . . about snotty waiters.

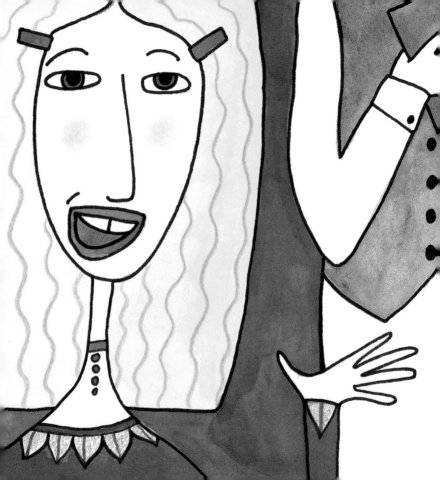

. . . about whether messenger bags
make me look "hippy."

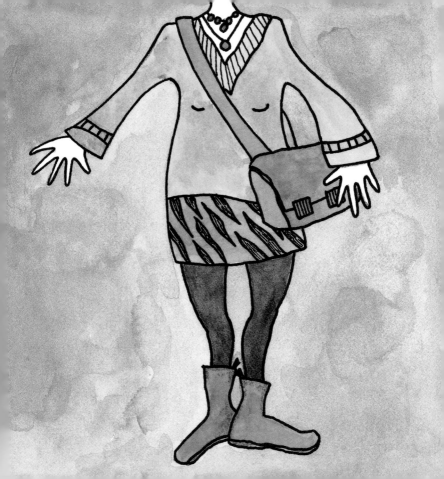

. . . about trying to be one of those
thong-butt babes!

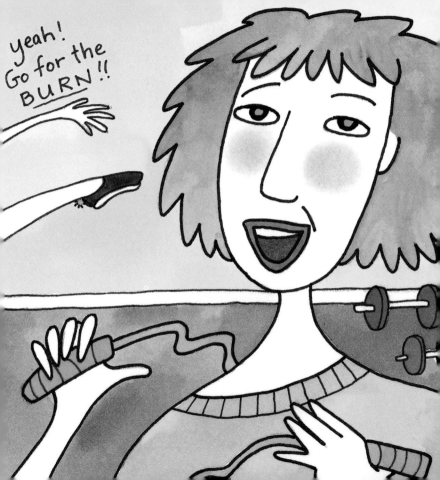

. . . about whether anyone notices
that I returned to the buffet. Again.

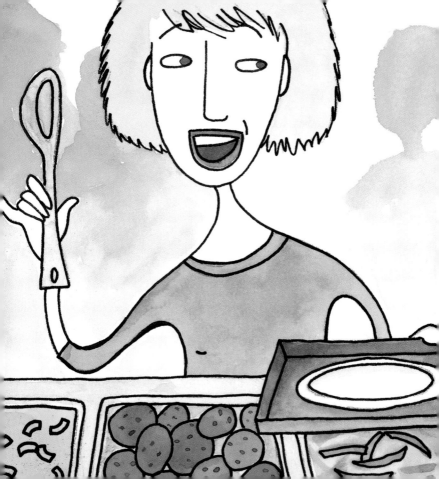

. . . about other people's hang-ups.

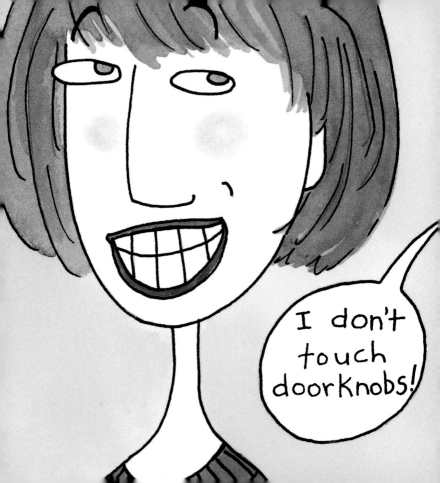

. . . about what the "popular" drink is.

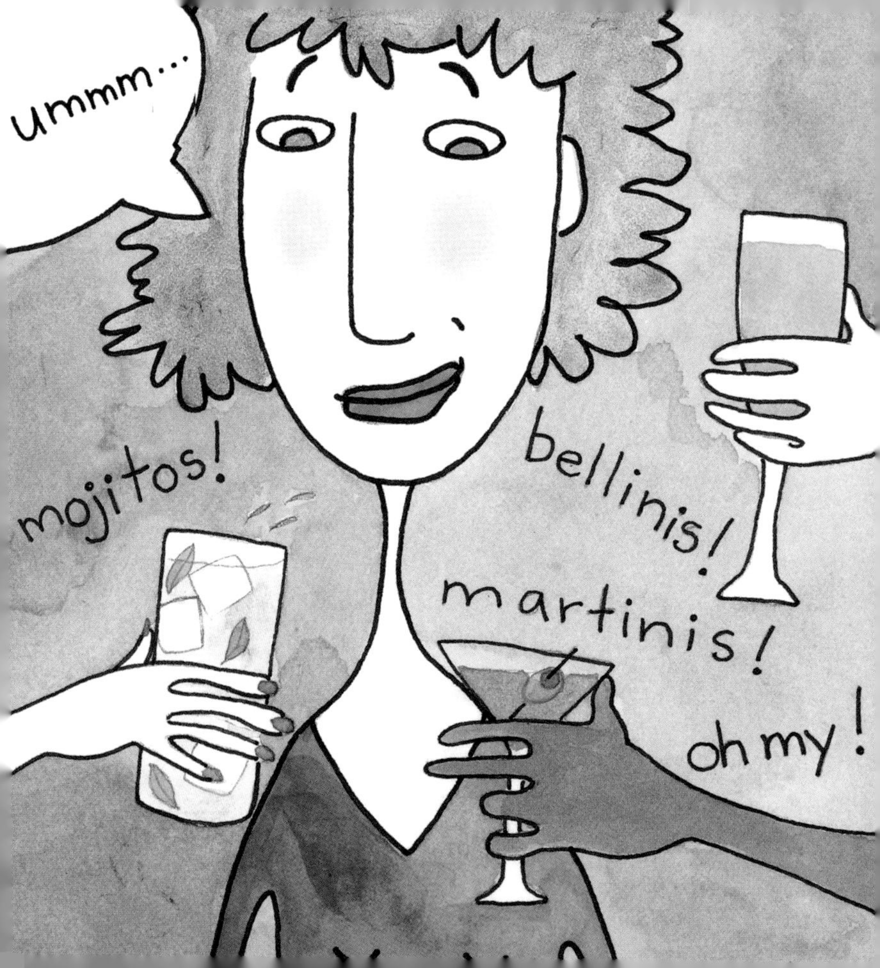
Ummm...
mojitos!
bellinis!
martinis!
oh my!

. . . about having too many purses.

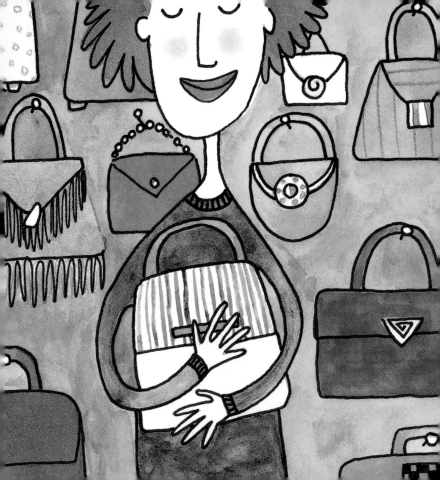

. . . about leaving up the
Christmas decor a little too long!

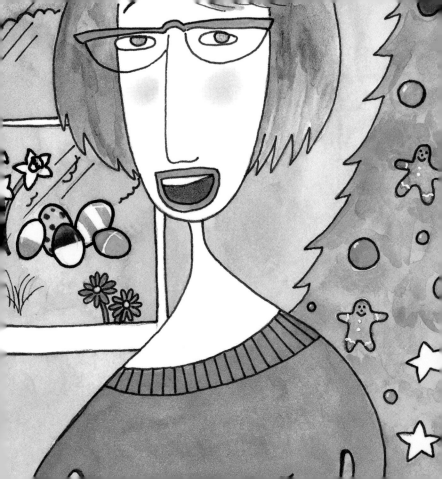

Linda Sue,

. . . about what's "IN" and what's "OUT"!

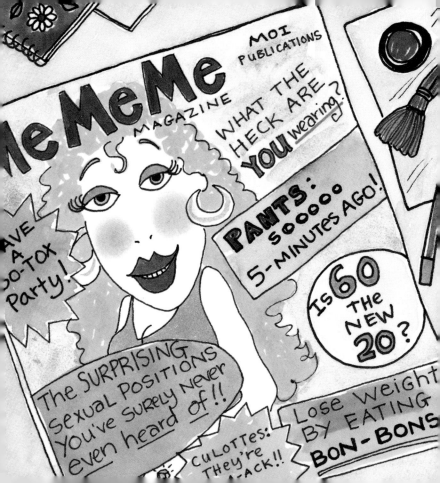

. . . about what "people" might
think if I got a tattoo!

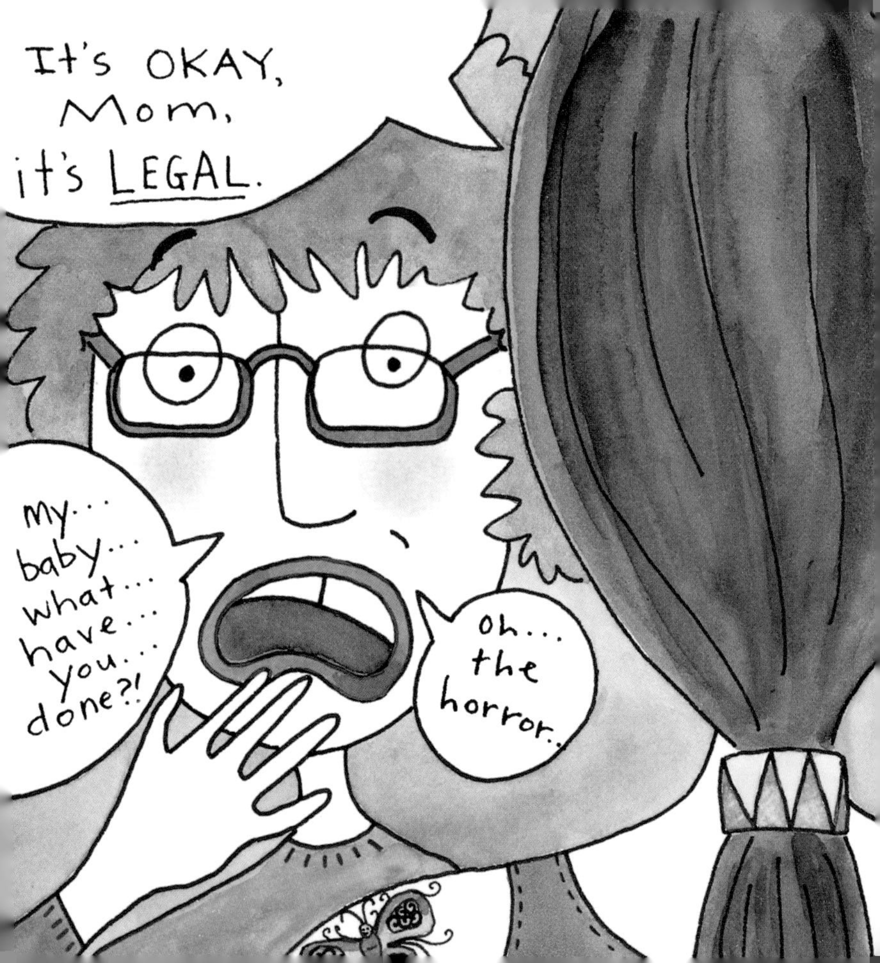
It's OKAY, Mom, it's LEGAL.
my... baby... what... have... you... done?!
oh... the horror...

. . . about when my vocabulary
takes a vacation!

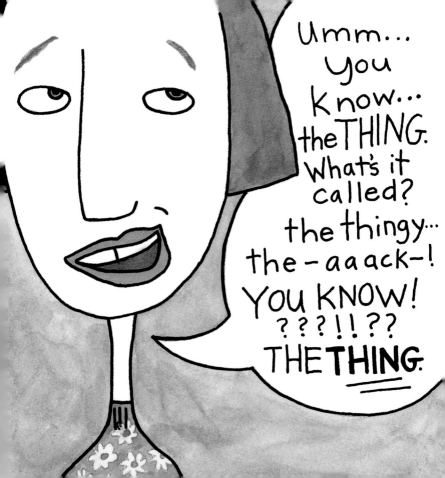

. . . about how much "anti-stress" articles stress me out!

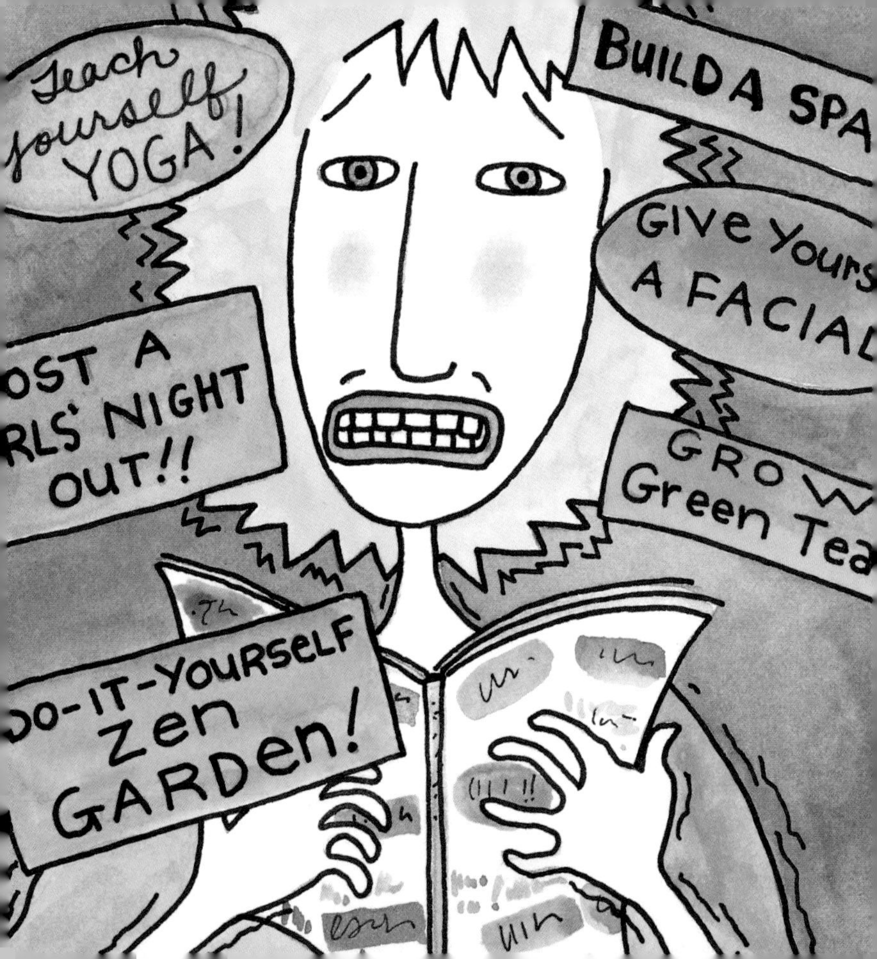
Teach yourself YOGA!
BUILD A SPA
Give Yours
A FACIAL
OST A
RLS' NIGHT
OUT!!
GROW
Green Tea
DO-IT-YOURSELF
Zen
GARDEN!

. . . about memory loss.

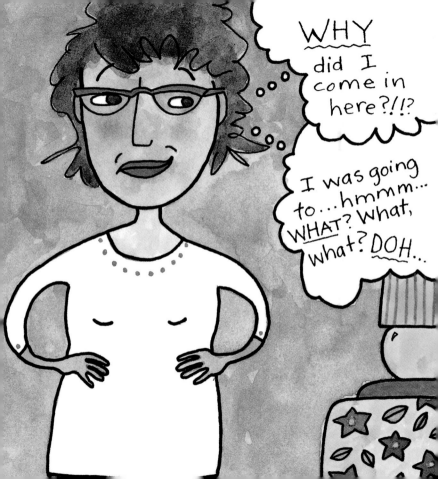

. . . about material goods!
Except for chocolate. Umm, chocolate
and shoes . . . Okay . . . chocolate,
shoes, and purses.

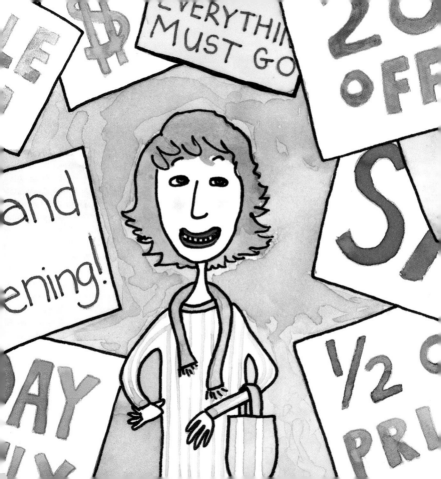

. . . about crazy bad-hair days.

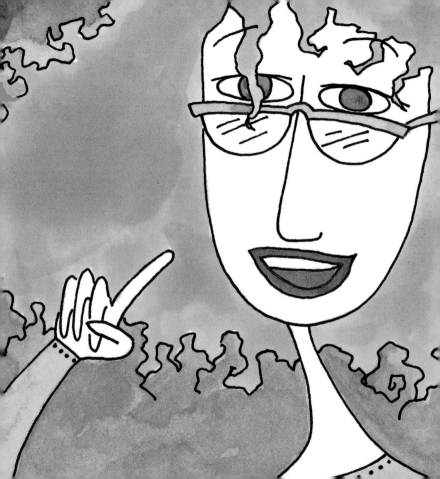

. . . about watching too many
episodes of *Sex and the City!*

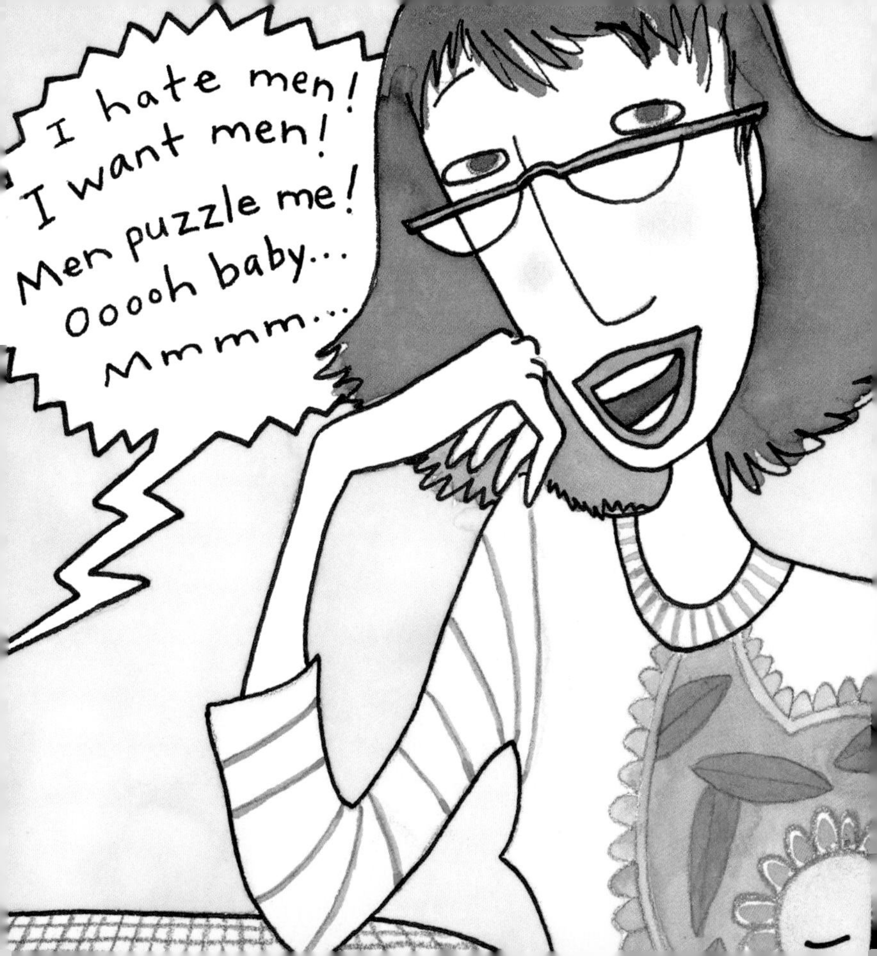

. . . about my butt being wider than
standard folding chairs.

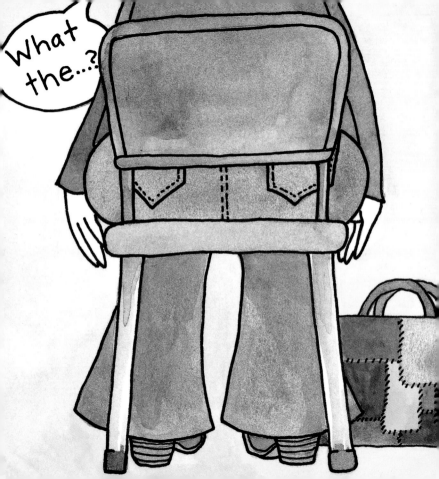

. . . about limiting my caffeine intake!

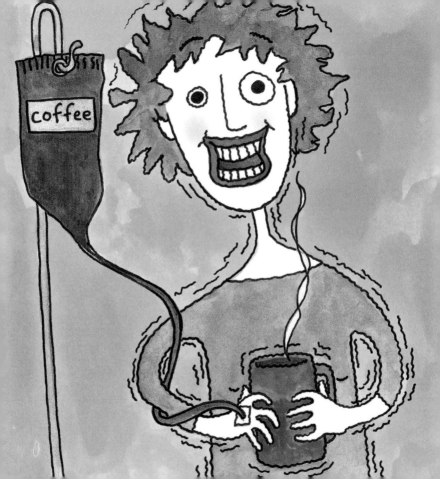

. . . about how much I spend
on wine and candles!

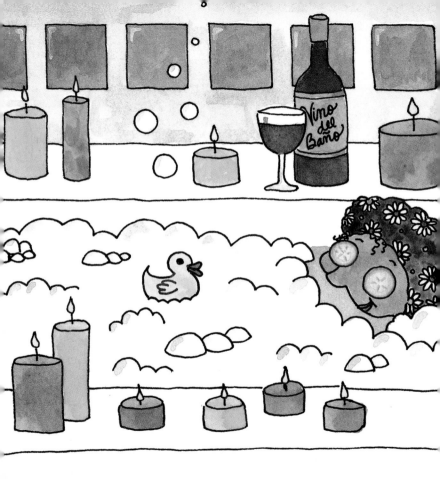

. . . about the fact that sometimes
"meditation" makes me angrier!

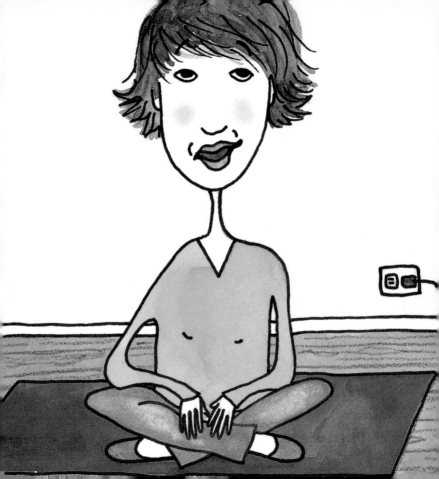